Thus I Became Stress Free
Oh, really?

B.Joshi Ph.D.

iUniverse, Inc.

New York   Bloomington

Thus I Became Stress Free

Oh, really?

iUniverse books may be ordered through booksellers or by contacting:

iUniverse
1663 Liberty Drive
Bloomington, IN 47403
www.iuniverse.com
1-800-Authors (1-800-288-4677)

*Because of the dynamic nature of the Internet, any Web addresses or links
contained in this book may have changed since publication and may no longer be
valid. The views expressed in this work are solely those of the author and do not
necessarily reflect the views of the publisher, and the publisher hereby disclaims
any responsibility for them.*

ISBN: 978-1-4401-1189-1 (sc)
ISBN: 978-1-4401-1190-7 (ebk)

Printed in the United States of America

iUniverse rev. date: 1/07/2009

Dedicated to my beloved BauJi,

Shri Harbans Rai Joshi

Preface

I had been hearing about stress and stress related problems for quite some time. I came across close friends and relatives who always talked of negative things about life and looked always burdened with some unknown problem. I could not realize the gravity until I started having loss of concentration in my work myself due to petty disturbing instances. While trying to figure out my problem, I suddenly recollected the instance of my childhood where problems were solved only by looking at those from a different angle. That instance is described in Chapter 1 of this book.

Most of my career has been administrative and managerial. I have run my own business, worked for government department, semi government company and private companies. I have lived in 10 different states in India, each state having vastly different culture. I have lived in Africa and presently I am living in U.S.A.

I hold Ph.D. in 'Coordination Chemistry'. This complements my capability to study, analyze and resolve a problem and then present its solution in an organized and effective manner. My expertise in managing stress is akin to anyone among the masses.

That I believe is a Big Plus because it makes my thinking, feeling, experiences, problems and solutions just like those for anybody else. That also means that analysis would be more effective and matching with the common person's requirement. I don't care what medical experts or other authorities on this subject say about medical treatments of this 'projected' complex problem. Yes, I call it 'projected' because the vested interests in multi trillion medical industry never support any treatment that does not take you to hospital. How could they? They have to have customers to sell new drugs on the discovery of which they have spent lot of money.

I have experienced lot of vicissitudes in life. Following some techniques from my past experiences and learning new techniques to handle stress made me feel so stress free, and it was so simple that I felt an urge to share it with the world. It would be worth my effort even if a few people could benefit from what I have learnt.

The instance quoted in the very first chapter of the book basically conveys everything this book is about. The detailed instance covered therein mainly re-enforces the expression 'The things change if you change the way you look at them'.

There are a number of depressing things those affect every one in day-to-day life. Everyone handles most of these problems successfully without really being aware of doing so. But many people don't handle the remaining problems in an organized way. This book is an effort to help reader handle the day-to-day problems without being stressed.

The book presents the reader with different scenarios with suggested approach. Potential sources of stress with related scenarios are included for easy grasp. You would come across a number of stress releasers those could help in a number of different situations. While explaining various stress-releasers, information about some important 'kriyas' of YOGA has been provided in detail. One chapter has been devoted to practical 'Hands-On' procedure to follow for achieving the desired results.

There are lot of interesting one liners used in the book to effectively bring the point home. One could read first chapter of this book under the link 'Chapter One' by visiting my website 'www.howibecamestressfree.com'.

Overall approach of this book is to help the reader minimize his/her stress level by conscious effort to achieve a wonderfully relaxed life style.

I must acknowledge my gratitude to my parents who have been source of my inspiration for main events of my life, including this book. I will be failing in my duty if I don't appreciate the cooperation I received from my wife, Asha Joshi, throughout this endeavor. My thanks are also due to Dr. Faik Nasser who was quite instrumental in bringing home many of the techniques described in this book. His contribution during discussions was really amazing.

Finally, I must thank the publisher, I Universe, which made it possible for me to bring this book to you.

Sd/

Balram Joshi

Contents

Chapter 1

Problems Solved!

That incident is quite vivid in my mind.

I was only 12 years of age and never even heard of stress problems. My father* was getting ready to go to the house of a common friend, Mr. Jindal. Mr. Jindal had invited a learned saint who would handle the problem of his devotees.

It was a fine Sunday morning. After reluctantly taking bath, I was sitting in our kitchen eating my typical favorite Punjabi breakfast that my mother was cooking on old styled charcoal grill. It was so delicious, as usual, I kept eating irrespective of my needs or even irrespective of space in my stomach. As I started feeling full, my mother asked me if I needed more. I reluctantly said no and she quickly wound up and went to get ready to give company to my father.

My father asked me to get ready so as to accompany them. I was in no mood to go anywhere on this rare holiday and requested

1

him to let me play. Immediately came a reprimand "You don't want to learn anything good. Babaji (as he called that saint) has solution to all problems". But I did not have any problems other than some spanking by schoolteachers now and then. Anyway I had to accompany my parents to join the congregation. Mr. Jindal's house was about half a mile from our home. We walked down to that place. There were about 35 to 40 people in the living room. Most of them were family friends. We found a place to sit right in front by the side of our neighbor, Sharma Ji. How I wished we could have sat somewhere in the rear.

The saint was speaking something about spirituality, *God and Karma* , which sometimes I would hear as part of sentences.

The saint, known as Baba Ji, was a very typical looking old wise man with flowing white beard. He was bearing some mysteriously calm smile on his face adding lot of grace to his personality. He was wearing a white *kurta* and white *dhoti*. He was sitting on an '*asan*' (a raised platform covered with cushioned mattress) with folded hands. Every now and then he would raise and wave his hands to emphasize some point and again would go back to his position of folded hands. Everybody, intermittently, was nodding his/her head as if to communicate their understanding and acceptance of the utterances of Baba Ji[1].

Suddenly I heard the saint addressing my father.

"Harivansh, I understand you have lot of problems".

(Although my father's first name was Harbans, Baba Ji used to address him like this only)

"Yes, Baba Ji", my father responded by standing up with folded hands.

---

1   *My father, Shri Harbans Rai Joshi, passed away in 1974. All this conversation is translated form Hindi.

"I can take care of most of them right now", said the saint.

"I am sure you would Baba Ji. I will be really grateful", my father said while bowing a little bit to the front.

"How many problems do you have? Can you give me a rough figure?"

"May be 20 to 25" my father did not want to look ignorant of his proclaimed problems.

"How many of these are due to unrealistic wishes?"

"None, Baba Ji"

"Do those keep you bothering all the time?"

"Yes, Baba Ji"

"OK, let me write those down on a piece of paper, umm…. The biggest problem on the top … go ahead, I am writing", said the saint while picking up a notebook and a pencil. Now was the turn of my father to start telling the problems. He was trying to start with a long list of problems but was little staggering. Finally he started.

"I don't have enough money for education of my children".

"Next".

"I have chronic back pain".

"Next".

"My wife keeps arguing with me on petty things".

"Next".

"My elder son does not have a good job".

By now my father had started really hesitating. He was noticing mischievous smile on the faces of his friends. But he bravely continued.

"My younger son is not good at studies".

"Next".

"My…my house needs major upgrading".

"Next".

"My boss creates problems for me in the office".

"Next".

"My neighbors are jealous of me".

"Next".

But before my father spoke further, Sharma Ji shouted

"That is my problem too".

Obviously my father had run out of his so-called long list of problems and was feeling embarrassed on his last stated problem. In order to escape from the unpleasant situation, he hurriedly said that he had no more problems.

"You said you had 20 to 25 problems. But as I count those on list, you have only 8 problems. So nearly 15 problems are already taken care just by making a list", mused Baba Ji. "And even out of 8 problems some are perceived problems and do not appear to be actual problems", continued Baba Ji.

By now every body was wondering whether they had any big problems they could not handle.

Then Baba Ji said, "Now Harivansh I want to ask you a few questions".

"Yes, Baba Ji", said my father submissively.

"Do you own a house?"

"Yes, Baba Ji"

"Are you married?"

"Yes, Baba Ji"

"Are your family members mentally sound?"

"Yes, Baba Ji".

"Do you have children?"

"Yes, Baba Ji".

"Do they have some chronic disease or physical disabilities?"

"No, Baba Ji"

"Do you have a job?"

"Yes, Baba Ji"

"Do you have any difficulty in feeding your family?"

"No, Baba Ji"

"Now, whether lack of any of these things I asked would be a bigger problem than any of the 8 problems you listed?"

"Definitely, Baba Ji"

"Harivansh, there are lot of similar things you have, lack of any one of which would be far bigger problem for you than the ones on your list".

"Yes, Baba Ji. I understand. Thanks a lot. I don't have any problem. I am fortunate to realize it".

Saying this, my father sat down with cheerful face.

Then Baba Ji asked, "Who else has lot of problems?" Nobody was ready to volunteer after seeing my father's list of problems. Then one devotee took the lead and said with folded hands, "Baba Ji you have enlightened us today. We unnecessarily keep thinking all the time that we are the cursed ones having biggest problems of the world".

"Yes, that's what I want all of you to realize. We should be thankful to the almighty for what He has given us and not complain for what He has not given us. That is the only way to have a peaceful happy life".

The saint then continued giving worldly advice as to how to be content and happy.

"You have to count your blessings, and not curses. Everybody in this world has some problem or the other. If you keep looking only at your curses, you can never be happy because everybody at any given time can find some deficiencies in life. Always be positive. God always helps you the way you want to help yourself. If you think negatively, that means you are trying to help yourself in a negative way. Same negative way would the God's help come. If you think positively, you would get helped by God in a positive way. Choice is yours". And many more wise sermons followed.

After sometime, *prasadam* was served and everybody left for his/her home after observing usual formalities.

I kept wondering about the existence of problems and solution to those problems.

I almost forgot about this incident until I had my own family and was in my late thirties.

———————————

Chapter 2

Identifying if You Are Stressed

First of all, let us try to know if you really have stress related problem or you just think you might have this problem.

Following are given a few questions for you to answer.

1. Do you have to make efforts to make yourself feel good? Do you keep searching for some extra agent to make you feel good?

2. Do you experience abnormal heartbeat some times during the day?

3. Do you find it hard to concentrate?

4. Do you experience tensed muscles?

5. Do you feel frequently irritated even on a normal question?

6. Whether you are unknowingly and unnecessarily rushing through daily routine items?

7. Whether you feel unexplained stiffness in your neck, back, shoulders, chest or stomach?

8. Do you have frequent unpleasant verbal exchanges for apparently petty things?

9. Whether unhappy events of distant past keep you bothered for more than 3 times everyday?

10. Are you too much worried about what is happening in the world? When you get up in the morning, do you have a feeling that whole world is bad and most of the happenings are negative?

11. Do you feel routinely fatigued even when there is no apparent reason for feeling tired, like excessive physical work or exercise?

12. Do you routinely face a situation where you feel uncomfortable about something but you can't figure it out?

13. Are you taking treatment for some chronic disease since a long time but not getting any improvement?

14. While sitting on a chair, do you keep tapping your feet involuntarily or keep twitching your fingers unknowingly?

15. Whether you feel your head heavy frequently without any apparent reason?

16. Whether you feel disturbance in your sleep?

If you answered 'Yes' to 6 or more of these questions you might be carrying more than average 'bad stress'.

———————————

Chapter 3

Stress – A Silent Killer!

Of course it does not need rocket science knowledge to know whether stress is bad. It is very simple to understand that why you should get rid of bad things. The very fact that you are reading this book means you already feel it to be important to lower your stress. There are good chances that you know only in general terms that it is good to have less stress, like it is always good to have less pain.

But just saying that a thing is bad would not have the same impact and not to the same extent on every person. You must be knowing many bad things but you may sometime not be able to gauge the extent of damage that bad things could inflict. Therefore you might not give them the importance or treatment they would deserve.

Another reason to know the details is that many of our ailments those might be related to stress, apparently, don't seem to be linked to it. You might keep taking treatments for those ailments without any benefits and keep wondering about the effectiveness of those treatments. You can very well figure out that if you keep getting the wrong diagnosis of any ailment, how much chances are there to cure it? That's why I thought helpful to devote one chapter to this topic so that potential impact of this problem could be properly comprehended.

Various reports have shown that stress could create diseases ranging from depression to early aging to reduced immune response and even cancer. It could disrupt normal family relations, could upset your productivity at job or school and even could lead to violent behavior.

"Psychology – An Introduction, By Benjamin B. Lahey, 7th Edition" states, inter alia, "*The extent to which stress is related to some of our most serious medical conditions was greatly underestimated until research dramatically altered our perceptions of our own health. Leading causes of death and disability such as heart disease and stroke are almost certainly linked to stress and immunity to infections is greatly affected by stress (Cohen and Williams, 1991). It is even probable that the link between stress and immunity extends to susceptibility of cancer (O'Leary, 1990; Taylor, 1986). In an era in which effective treatments are available for a wide variety of infectious diseases, the major killers are stress related diseases and cancer.*"

William Kornblum and Joseph Julien's "Social Problems" (10th Edition) contains many startling facts on the effects caused by stress. It mentions: "*Some researchers are convinced that each of us carries a personal time table for aging within our cells, a time table that is controlled by our genes. Others believe that other factors are also involved. The role of stress is particularly important. One of the main salient age-related changes is the decline in homeostatic capacity – the ability to tolerate stress. This makes older people more susceptible to stress and it takes longer to return to normal after being exposed to stressful situation.*

The reduced capacity to cope with stress is a result of primary aging; stress itself is an agent of secondary aging. Together they may be responsible for many of the illnesses that plague the elderly...~.......
Studies have demonstrated that such illnesses as leukemia, cancer and heart disease often strike in the wake of stress producing life changes (Rowe J.W., & R.L.Kahn, 1998, Successful Aging)".

Readers Digest, July 2005, on page 49 has quoted from 'Research presented at the AHA 45th Annual Conference on cardiovascular Disease, Epidemiology and Prevention under the subtitle. 'Relax Your Heart' – *"Doctors recommend that people with heart disease exercise to reduce their risk of heart attack. But managing stress may be just as important, say researchers at Duke University Medical Center."* They further made study on 134 heart patients and concluded *"This study adds to what we already know, says cardiologist Nieca Goldberg of the American Heart Association: we need a comprehensive program of diet, exercise and stress management to achieve complete heart health."*

Bottomline Health in vol.19, number 6, June 2005, page 3 under the heading 'Don't Ignore These Dangerous Symptoms' mentions this about depression, *"This mental health problem is as common in older adults as in younger people, and the associated risk for suicide is highest among older white men."*

Gary Small, MD, University Of California at Los Angels, while writing in 'Bottomline Health Vol. 19, number 5, May 2005 on page 8, recommended cutting stress for improving memory, as one of the several points. It further mentions, *"The hormones triggered by stress, most prominently cortisol, have a toxic effect on the brain, in general, and memory in particular. Over time, the effect of stress on blood pressure and arterial disease will reduce cerebral circulation, which impairs brain functioning and raises stroke risk."*

Lifepositive.com mentions in a report in August 2005, *"Medically it has been established that chronic symptoms of anxiety and stress* can crumble our body's immune system. Irrespective of the nature of causes of stress – real or perceived – our subconscious mind reacts with the same body response by releasing stress hormones equal to the degree of our fear, worry or sense of threat. It brings about changes in the body's biochemical state with extra epinephrine and other adrenal steroids such as hydrocortisone in the blood stream. It also induces increased palpitation and blood pressure in the body with mental manifestations such as anger, worry, fear or aggression. In short, stress creates anomalies in our body's homeostasis.

When the extra chemicals in our blood stream don't get used up or the stress situation persists, it makes our body prone to mental and physical illness. ..~.....~...New medical research has established that prenatal stress could significantly influence development of the brain and organization of behavior in fetus. Researchers explain that because stress affects many of the body systems – nervous, cardiovascular, endocrine and immune- there is a good reason to believe that severe emotional stress could cause defects in the fetus, especially during first trimester of pregnancy when development occurs at faster rate..~..~..

Aging is a natural and gradual process, except under extreme circumstances such as stress or grief. The constant stressors or stress conditions result in a loss in neural and hormonal balance. The loss in balance will cause increased oxidative damage accelerating aging in our body...~..~..

The study suggests that chronic stress may accelerate hippocampal deterioration leading to accelerated physical and brain aging....~...~..

Stress is known to worsen many immune related medical conditions, including diabetes. Cortisol produced during stress may suppress the body's immune response increasing susceptibility to infectious diseases...~..~...

In severe stress conditions blood supply to stomach is restricted, hampering normal digestive function. Also the function of the entire intestine is controlled partly by the nervous system, which in turn is directly affected by stress. These conditions including one's diet during stress can offset gastrointestinal disorders such as ulcer or irritable bowel syndrome....~..~...

It is now established that stress, cognitive appraisal, coping and migraine are reciprocally related. Stress is detrimental to the body and can cause back pains, neck pains and headache....~..~...

A path breaking research conducted in early 90's showed stress induced reduction in T-Lymphocytes (white blood cells that destroy cancer cells) in the human body leading to an increase in metastasis. A later study on women suffering from breast cancer reestablished the previous findings and confirmed the fact that stressors cause lowest levels of natural-killer-cell activity in the body....~...~..

Chronic stress induced homeostasis changes and immune reduction, tends to affect the balance between oxidants and antioxidants in the body. Many ongoing studies have found that alteration in this balance in favor of oxidants may result in pathological responses causing functional disorders and diseases such as cancer and Alzheimer's disease. It can also accelerate the aging process, for oxidation increases electronegative constituents in body molecules mutilating the 'blue print' of the cells. Multiplication of distorted cells can set in cancer."

In a report on livescience.com by Jeanna Bryner titled "Skin disorders linked to stress" the effects of stress have been shown to decrease cell growth and inhibit differentiation in to skin cells.

Thus you see above that there is almost no serious disease that is not caused or aggravated by stress.

The purpose of course is not to scare you. It is rather to apprise you about the serious potential consequences of bad stress.

Another point to be noted is that in the event of having any of these diseases, the diagnosis should include the possibility of contribution by stress.

Let us next try to differentiate between right type and wrong type of stress.

———————————

Chapter 4

Managing Stress

Good Stress – Bad Stress

You might have noticed a benign question on the title - Oh, really? Let me explain. The question is not meant to communicate the impression that it is not possible to become stress free. What it means is that being stress free is not a static state, because our life is not static. Our life is dynamic and so is our state of mind. And stress is directly related to the state of mind. Mind keeps getting affected day in and day out by numerous ongoing incidents. So, even if you manage to become stress free today does not ensure you to be stress free the next day unless you again use the methodology you used today to become stress free. With practice you would be able to continuously stay in a state of least stress.

That leads to another very important question. Whether it is good to be free of all types of stress? And whether all types of stress are bad? I would say "not really".

Many things you accomplish won't be possible without certain degree of stress. In the total absence of stress, life would not stay as interesting, or even as productive, or as challenging. Many studies have shown that under controlled conditions, or the adrenaline in moderate doses, helps you to achieve what you would not achieve with totally stress free mind. Stress levels in the middle range, not very low, not very high, actually are known to improve performance by improving your alertness. At moderate levels, the increased blood flow to the brain helps improve brain's performance, which further helps you to remain alert and better focused. You must have come across reports that suggest that senior people who undertake challenging mental exercises like solving crosswords or solving other puzzles have less chances of getting Alzheimer's. To differentiate between this stress and other stress, I like to call it 'Good Stress'

Stress broadly could be divided into two types – 'Good Stress' and 'Bad Stress'. This I would compare with 'Good Cholesterol' and 'Bad Cholesterol'. We want to get rid of bad cholesterol but want a healthy dose of good cholesterol. Similarly, we want to get free of 'Bad Stress' and need moderate dose of 'Good Stress' in certain circumstances.

May be there is another way of saying it

- Stress, which leads to depression of mind, is 'bad' type of stress.

- Stress, which is affecting only our anxiety in a positive way and ends up in motivating the process we are trying to complete and helps to concentrate on the work in hand, is 'good' type of stress.

There are many instances where stress helps you in a positive way in our day-to-day life. On many occasions you might have noticed that when you have lot of work pending due to be completed in a short time, you are under some sort of stress to meet the deadline. Your output at that time far exceeds your output in normal circumstances. Sometimes stress helps you meet certain challenges in life. Rather sometimes you take up a challenge, more often than not, because your mind is provoked by certain circumstances to consider meeting that challenge equivalent to protecting our respect or image or family's honor. That provocation of mind is having another manifestation of stress. In all these cases it was 'good stress' at work. You would come across some interesting instances for upsides of moderate stress later.

If you combine this argument with the earlier stated presentation about static and dynamic stress, your goal settles down to manage bad stress and not being stress free. Therefore it would be fair to say that 'we don't want to be free of all stress. It would bring us best results if we could manage our stress'.

In the subsequent chapters we would try to deal with this 'bad' type of stress. We would try to elaborate how to manage bad stress. I may remind you that this book is not about solving problems. All this book deals with is managing stress that we get as a result of problems. Of course with a handle on stress you would be able to handle the problems also more effectively.

Chapter 5

Analyses and Sources of Stress

In the last chapter you have seen that it is the bad stress that we are trying to manage and that we are not trying to be totally free of stress because that would be nearly unachievable. It is positively possible to develop a system, put controls in place and have an attitude to control stress in any and every situation.

Here we are not talking something with physical form or something material. We are talking something that is in our mind. Stress could be seen as absence of specific body response to different thoughts created by association with differently perceived incidents.

Stress to the mind could be due to one factor or combination of factors. Stress could be characterized as intangible demands made on our system by various incidents/thoughts. Stress can also be explained in terms of chemical changes in our body wrought by thought processes generated by our day-to-day exposure to specific and non-specific incidents. Medical experts could provide many complicated explanations and prescribe many drugs/ therapies to cure it. But what we are talking here is simplest of the simplest and durable ways how a common person could take care of this seemingly complex problem. A little reminder here, I think, would be in order.

This book is not about solving problems. It is about managing stress during the time of facing and handling problems and to control our state of mind that we are in because of those problems.

Let us try next to answer whether stress is simple or complex. This all depends on the individual handling it, though that does not mean that all sources of stress are of the same gravity. What I mean to say is that our approach could make a big difference in resultant gravity of stress attached with any problem. More you think it to be difficult, more difficult it would be to handle. In that case handling stress itself would be stressful.

Before going into details of various *'common man's'* reasons of stress, it might be relevant, and may be helpful here, to have a little promenade in the gardens of science. We will cast a bit light here and there and move to examples from our life.

The joy to the body after a long walk is indescribable. One might feel pain all over one's muscles, but there are very special euphoria waves all over you. Scientists looked in to the mechanism of this feeling. They found that some chemicals secreted or were generated by the cells (de novo synthesis) in the blood of those who had a long walk. These compounds are identified as endomorphins. They are small chain of amino acids. It has been established that these compounds do impact favorably in relieving stress and produce a state of wellbeing. This feeling is like the way you feel when you stretch your limbs after sitting for long in one position. You might have noticed such stretching being done by pet animals in your house. It gives same refreshing feeling that you get after body massage, though to a lesser degree. Why do you feel good when somebody strokes the hands over you with gentle pressure on certain spots all over your body? The person who provided biochemical explanation to this phenomenon earned Nobel Prize in medicine. Part of the explanation given is very simple. The cells of our body make some specific molecules in extremely small amount. These molecules are called nitric oxide. These cause stiff muscles and vessels to dilate, loosen them up, so that more blood could be pumped into them. This results in good feeling.

Sanskrit word for happiness or fulfilling joy is '*anand*'.

It was found that a chemical that belongs to the family of amides and also an active ingredient of marijuana is the reason behind people getting hooked on to marijuana. It is in this context, may be, that scientists named this chemical '*anandamide*' (anand+amide), also known as arachidonoylethanolamide (AEA). It is also interesting to know that same chemical is also present in chocolate. Some attribute this chemical the responsibility of increasing the desire to eat more carbohydrates. No wonder people under stress tend to eat more of such foods.

Enough of this science of stress! Let us get back to our links of stress to our daily life incidents and simple ways to look at it. Please understand that accounts mentioned hereafter are only some glimpses. As we move on in our mission, further relevant parts will be added.

Referring stress to look at in simple ways is not meant to underestimate this universally prevalent problem. Also all reasons contributing to stress might not be as simple as might be concluded form the instance given in chapter one. The purpose of quoting that instance, I emphasize, was only to show how your thinking could make all that big difference in your life. And again, way of thinking can work wonders with our ultimate target – stress. There could be benign and not-so-benign factors contributing to stress. There could be lot many reasons for your stress. Everybody would not have same reasons for his/her stress nor same reasons would influence everybody in the same way, but everybody can handle his/her factors leading to stress in the same systematic way to achieve desired results.

What are different sources of stress?

To make an exhaustive list of reasons contributing to, or causing stress is impossible as well as undesirable, and of very limited use since each individual is having different personality and different approach to handle different problems. Further, a reason of stress for somebody might be a motivating stress (good stress) for someone else. There is a popular saying "One's loss is somebody else's gain". So the same event could bring joy to some and grief to others. Another reason for not attempting to make a list of all the situations causing stress is to keep this book simple, readable and understandable.

The purpose of this book is not to make the reader know all the situations causing stress, but to try to develop a way to handle every possible situation he/she faces.

All of us face numerous instances everyday those could result in creating stress if not handled properly. As a matter of fact, each one of us is already successfully handling many such situations everyday. The proof for that is that if those situations were not handled properly and would have been allowed to develop into stress, each one of us would have a big load of stress everyday to unmanageable extent. It would have been almost impossible to survive.

Keeping that in mind, the approach in this book is to categorize potential stress creators into general groups. The purpose, again, is not to cover everything under the sun, but to illustrate, hands-on, as to how to tackle them.

The main categories identified are:

1. Family

2. Spouse

3. Friends and neighbors

4. Workplace

5. Finances

6. Politics

7. Sports

8. Religion

9. Health Concerning

10. Legal

11. Fate related

12. Expectations

13. Ambitions

14. Materialism

Before demonstrating each category by example, little description of each category would be useful.

1. **Family:** Family related stressful situations become generally more dominant when you are married and having children. Other than that it could be your relationship with your parents. Though 1st and 2nd cousins and their families could be a potential source of awful situations, but those are relatively

less stress causing because you don't have to face those on daily basis and there is always a chance for you to opt out.

2. **Spouse:** Though this category is very similar to the first category, it has a separate importance of its own because of the special relationship this category enjoys. This creates unique situations where even a smile or quiet face could be possibly meaning a lot with regard to releasing or creating tension. Implications of this relationship are dynamic in nature, ever changing with time.

3. **Friends and neighbors:** Friends and neighbors generally create a transitional situation. Very few friends stick with you for life. Here filtration process is always in operation. Only those are left with whom you feel comfortable. There is not much stress creation unless your friend himself faces some situations. Neighbors, unless they are creating some physical problems, could be handled easily, just by avoiding.

4. **Workplace:** This could be a major cause of stress in many individuals since a major portion of your active time you spend at work. Not only it is because of this time that you spend over there, strain could be the result of your actions or inactions at work that could affect your life materially. Sometimes you are in a situation you don't want to face but neither can you run away from it. Not only that, you keep thinking or talking about workplace events even after you leave your workplace. There have been quite a few instances that an employee went to the extent of hurting his coworkers and hurting himself.

At the same time, if you look at it from a different angle, workplace related stress is not that difficult to manage because there is no need or use of bringing negative emotions from there to home. It is further explained later in this chapter.

5. **Finances:** Finance related stress could be a big source of stress to lot many people. Usually mismanaging finances is one of the most common factor contributing to financial troubles. Many people try to avoid the problems created by this category by simply not paying systematic attention to it. This leads to even bigger problem. Most common in this category is mounting debt that once created and not properly managed puts one in a vicious cycle. Low income could sometimes create this problem but is not always the reason for this situation. Mostly it is mismanagement and not having the will to deal it heads on.

6. **Politics:** Political environment in the city, workplace or country could stir lot of emotions but constitutes very low cause of stress unless you involve yourself too much in this. In any case it is transitory in nature except for the people who have political careers.

7. **Sports:** Sports again could make a temporary cause of stress to some fans, similar to the above category.

8. **Religion:** Religion for most people is stress releaser rather than stress creator. The fabric of society itself is woven around it. It is true for all religions. Some even believe that some wise people, to keep the wheel of society running smoothly, invented religion. Whatever be the truth in their thinking, my personal belief is that lack of trust in some superpower makes it difficult to handle many situations in life and has the potential of stress creation on frequent basis. Some specific customs attached with practicing of religion could create a problem when somebody close to you is too scrupulous in following literally some outdated strict rituals that you consider as irrelevant and/or tedious.

9. **Health Concerning:** Physical problems could be a big source and good reason for continuous stress depending on nature

and costs of the problem. In some cases, interestingly, the reverse could be true. Those problems might have reached the level of this aggravation because of stress.

10. **Legal:** Legal entanglements could make anybody's life mess and could be a continuous source of stress particularly its aftermaths in the event of unfavorable results.

11. **Fate Related:** Stressful conditions also could be attributed to our destiny such as having grief in family or many other situations we find ourselves in.

12. **Expectations:** This category is a routine contributor of stress but at the same time most easily manageable. Any results those don't match our expectations, generally, lead to stress.

13. **Ambitions:** Here is a category which is very essential for reaching high goals but at the same time, if unrealistic, makes you stressed even after achieving good level of success. You would be surprised by some examples quoted in the suggested solution section of this category.

14. **Materialism:** Everybody wants to own latest cars or other gadgets. But everybody can't afford everything. Strong wish to have some goodies not affordable in your means is a potential cause leading to stress.

Each of these categories, though not totally independent from each other could have thousands of scenarios in our daily life. You are dealing with these scenarios daily without realizing that you are already handling most of these potential stress creators without even realizing this. How do I say that? You know that by end of the day and by the end of the week you don't have hundreds or even tens of problems on your mind. You have only a few concerns on your mind, mostly.

What does it mean? It can mean only one thing that your mind did the best for you, that is, did not come under stress because of most of those events.

Bingo, here you are already doing what you should be consciously doing for remaining concerns on your mind.

Only the bigger stress creators remain in our mind. So you have really much smaller problem than you thought. Again, remember, top problems would be different for different people depending on personal priorities.

How to make conscious effort to handle stress in systematic way would be shown in later chapter. But for taking full advantage from that procedure, it would, in my view, do immense help to attempt to tackle one specific situation of each category.

Category 1

Problem 1:

Your son is not doing well in school.

Suggested Approach:

The very definition of 'not doing well' must be examined first. He is 'not doing well' compared to what? Compared to your expectations or compared to other students of his class? You know what – consider this. What would you have thought about Bill Gates' education in his college years? What would you have thought about academic record of President George W. Bush? So, the point is that first you have to see what is the standard you are applying for 'not doing well'.

If you are comparing to other students, compare not only with better students, compare with worse students as well.

By the way, how would you feel if your spouse compares you with other spouses in your circle?

Everybody is different having different skills and different qualities.

You are doing your job perfectly if you are providing the guidance (not comparing or forcing) and necessary means for your child's education.

Think for a moment this way. Consider yourself a tool through which God is passing on necessary means for your child to his own destiny.

If you could take the above said approach, you would definitely feel better thus reducing your stress level from this 'problem'.

Category 2

Problem 2:

Your husband has all the time in the world to watch football match or reading newspaper, but he does not have any time to help you in the kitchen whereas both of you are working full time jobs.

OR

Your wife keeps complaining about shortage of time when asked to make any dish but has all the time to spend in a department store.

Suggested Approach:

These small irritants could turn in to a big problem if not tackled in time. These thoughts could be nagging their minds and they could go to the extent of concluding that his/her partner does not care for her/him. Usually bigger conflicts start from very small irritants. Both of them need look at these thoughts with a different approach. Here you are dealing with two different individuals who have different tastes, or to be specific, different priorities. None of the acts under discussion, to say the least, are wrong. Rather those are normal acts with respect to each individual. Further, when you talk of persons of different genders, chances of having different priorities further go up. You cannot, and should not, try to match each other's priorities because that would not work on long-term basis. There are many instances quoted in literature about the behavior expectations of different genders, one being the book titled "Men are from Mars, Women are from Venus". I am not trying to apply logic of this title to this instance. I am merely trying to emphasize that both individuals are behaving in a normal way, the only difference being their interpretation about each other's actions. If they try to see from this angle, their chances of thinking and acting harmoniously would improve causing stress reduction.

Problem 3

Your girlfriend did not remember your birthday whereas you had thrown a grand treat at her birthday.

Suggested approach

On the face of it, it makes one to conclude that the girlfriend was not caring for your important days whereas you were doing more than average on her similar event. Or, you might conclude that she is not giving that much attention to details after lapse of some years of relationship as much she used to give in the beginning. This inference could again become a genuine irritant between the two. Here the dominant cause at play is 'expectation', also dealt as a separate category later.

Here, after giving extra importance on her birthday, you expect equal or better importance on a similar occasion for yourself. You took the initiative to please her in a specific way related to that particular occasion. When similar occasion came for you, you were expecting her to respond in equal or better way. But you had just done what you considered right to make her happy. Had you not opened an 'account' for your good deeds to be matched by her, you would not have felt bad. She just took his attempt to make her happy as a normal thing and not as some 'account' for repaying. It is quite possible that on some other occasion, you would have hurt her expectations in the same way but not realizing the same. So the problem could be traced to 'expectations' and not intentions.

If they realize this, there should be no problem.

Category 3

Problem 4:

My friend always complains to me for not giving him ride when he needs, whereas fact is just the opposite.

Suggested Approach:

You know what the truth is. It is only your friend's perception that he does more for you. It should be simple to make him see reason. Make a record of such events for some length of time and when such discussion comes up show that to him. If he complains even after that, then it is his problem and don't let it become your problem. Another conclusion could be that he is not a reasonable person and sincere friend, and therefore thoughts of his feeling bad should not bother you. He might not deserve your attention to the extent that his feelings should disturb you. Once you feel in yourself justified, your connected stress should also minimize.

Category 4

Problem 5:

Your boss always nitpicks on you on every small thing whereas he chooses to ignore big mistakes by your coworkers.

Suggested approach:

There could be various real reasons for your boss to behave like you perceive him to be behaving. This could be real or a case of insufficient information. But to deal it in general way, approach has to be objective. There could be different solutions to this problem depending upon personal characteristics of all involved, environments and circumstances. But here we are not trying to change the behavior of your boss or any body else. What your objective, in our scope, is to manage your stress, which in turn could help you improve the situation in more than one way for all concerned, including your family.

First step in this direction would be:

Do not bring problem home.

Look at it this way.

You probably work for 40 hours a week out of 168 hours that make a week (24x7=168). That means your time at work is only 23.8% of your total time. Counting holidays and vacation time would make even less than 23.8%. That means during the balance 76.2% of your total time nobody could nitpick on you. So at least 76.2% of your time, your mind should not be disturbed. There is a high possibility that even at work it is not happening all the time or not even every day. The few times such event occur, you might be carrying it in your mind even during rest of your quality time. This also might be leading to further aggravating the situation when such event occurs the next time. Chances are that you would over-react to your boss's action because you already carry a biased mind resulting from the last event. Is it not possible that even during last such occurrence your mind was already biased?

Take one thing at a time. May be the situation is worsening because your boss finds you overreacting on small things. Give it a break. Start thinking about your own physique and the quality time your family deserves with you. Even if your analysis in the first place is right, your balanced approach could make the things better for you, your family and even at office. And the other goal - stress would come down.

Let me also mention that there is another approach that surely works but some may not like it due to their personality. That approach is – become thick skinned. As long as you are not materially harmed, don't bother.

Category 5

Problem 6:

My credit card payments are ever increasing even though I pay 'minimum due' on regular basis.

Suggested approach:

This category is very common and very potential stress contributor. In this case stress is directly linked to the problem and is recurring in nature. It is different here. The problem needs to be handled to handle the stress. Of course for doing that stress releaser number 4 of Chapter 6, namely, 'If you keep doing whatever you have been doing, you would keep getting the results you had been getting', would be useful. Also remember the rule that 'better handling of stress would not only release your stress, it would also prepare you to handle the problem in more efficient way'. Though it would be important to change the attitude to tackle this problem, that alone is not going to be sufficient. You have to get out of this vicious cycle. Hard decisions need be taken. The problem itself has to be attacked.

First, it is good that at least you recognize this to be a problem, because unless you recognize something as a problem, you are not going to attempt find its solution. Ignoring any problem makes it worse. In most cases it would not be insurmountable problem. The solution – *Financial Discipline! Financial discipline! Financial discipline!* Financial discipline though is good at all times, but in the current situation, it is a must.

In case you are not confident of handling this situation yourself, seek help from somebody knowledgeable. I believe what it really needs is just plain common sense.

Here are a few suggestions.

- Make a detailed list of your income.

- Make a detailed list of your expenses. It may take some time to include all expenses in this list since some expenses are periodic and some non-recurring. Going through your credit card bills for last one year may be a good start.

- Calculate periodic expenses on per month basis (like auto insurance is paid 6 monthly, home insurance is paid annually, auto repairs may be incurred at irregular periods, etc.). Remember, paying late fees for any payment and interest is also an expense.

- Rearrange this list in the order of priority, most important being at the top. Remember paying off credit is one of the most important things. Show the expense against each item. Expense against credit card payments has to be calculated in a way so that your monthly balance even after interest expense would go down.

- Enter your monthly income in the calculator and start deducting amount of each item from the expense list starting from top. When calculator shows negative amount, STOP! The last item you entered is not permissible. If you think that there are still some items that are essential and not yet entered, you might have to redo your list and change the order of priorities. Or you have the alternative of increasing your income by taking some additional part time job.

- After you have done the above exercise, you have to take a hard decision to delete the items you could not enter in to the calculator from your list and from your life, hopefully, temporarily until you have taken care of this debt problem.

In addition you have to pay attention to the following.

- Never be late in sending 'minimum due'.

- Never send only 'minimum due'. Send more to the extent your budget allows.

- Consolidate higher interest rate carrying balances in to a low rate loan (home equity loan in most cases).

- Consider selling newer car, and buying reasonably old car having better fuel efficiency and the one worth low auto insurance.

- Consider 'no fault' insurance or the lowest level of

insurance with higher deductible.

- Reduce the frequency of vacations, movies, concerts, game watching and the like.

- Try to make meals at home and carry lunch and drinks to your work. This also provides you healthy food in addition to cutting costs.

- Never buy any item on impulse. Make a list of the items you need before going to a store. Stick to the list.

- Try shopping at discount stores. Sometimes fairly nice condition items are available at thrifty stores.

- Buy generic brands of medicines.

There are a lot of different steps you could take, but the order of those steps would depend on individual situations and after critically evaluating each expense.

One thing of course is certain and applicable to all – write down the expenses and income.

Once you do this exercise, you would start seeing that there is a plan available and that itself would calm your anxiety.

Category 6

Problem 7:

In your view the reelection of President George W. Bush was wrong.

Suggested Approach:

We live in democracy and we are proud of that. Every individual has a right to make his own opinion. The very fact that majority of people chose to vote for him shows that majority of people do not have the same opinion as you. It is better to come down to reality. It won't hurt. Moreover, as the time passes, new evaluations keep evolving.

Thinking on these lines would make you feel better.

Category 7

Problem 9:

Pistons were playing better, but Cavaliers won the NBA championship.

Suggested Approach:

This appears to be the statement form 'Pistons' fan. The word fan itself is from the family of word 'fanatic'. That means a 'fan' would likely think in a biased way favoring the team he wants to win. Neutrally considered, 'let the better team win'. Then of course, every body has his lucky days.

Category 8

Problem 9:

Your spouse does not go to church every Sunday.

Suggested Approach:

So what? Going to Church every Sunday is your top priority, not her! It is not necessary that your spouse would have the same priorities. There might be lot of things your spouse might like you to do but you might be putting those away. Try to respect your spouse's priorities because mutual respect for each other's characteristics is the very foundation of a successful marriage.

Even if some member in your family wants to practice a different religion, the best way to avoid bad situation is to understand and try to make the other person understand in a logical and rational manner. By trying to force your beliefs on other person, you might be pushing him to the corner that might generate reaction with worse results. Mutual respect is a MUST in case of religious beliefs.

If you ever had a chance to read the religious books or to listen to wise people of your community, every religion teaches you to

- Consider all creatures as part of the Almighty Himself.

- Consider everybody equal.

- Avoid judging others.

- Avoid assigning motives to others' actions.

- Be kind to everyone.

- Have mutual respect for everyone.' And so on.

If you cannot practice these things in your own family and cannot have mutual respect, how much you think you are justified in pushing others in the name of religion.

Looked from this angle might make you feel more sober towards your spouse's religious leanings/actions.

Category 9

Problem 10:

You have chronic asthma and cannot enjoy life like others do.

Suggested approach:

Let me first point out: 'Having stress further aggravates asthma'. Chances are that your level of asthmatic problem would have been less severe if you had handled your stress better. Even now if you try appropriate 'stress releaser' suiting to your temperament and routine from next couple of chapters, your asthmatic problem would be reduced.

The problem you feel is that you cannot enjoy various activities others are enjoying because of asthma. Dump this comparison and ask yourself 'how much can I enjoy even with this problem?' Just to make a point if I start brooding over the thoughts that I can not play base ball as good as Semi Sosa, or I can not play tennis as good as Roger Federer, would that bode good for me? Should that be a good reason for me to feel miserable? So the point is that even without this problem, there would always be somebody enjoying life more than you. That should settle the question of comparing with others. Comparison could help you if you take motivation to recover from the comparison. Once you put yourself in that positive frame of mind, you would definitely find your problem alleviated.

Category 10

Problem 11:

Your brother has gone to court over division of your ancestral property and the case has been going on for two years.

Suggested approach:

You are already doing what you can do, that is, fighting the case in court. Possibly you have already attempted to settle it out of court by trying to make your brother see reason. Possibly, your friends and relatives have also already weighed in to resolve the problem. Moreover, you don't have control over the outcome of this case. The anxiety you face with the thought of different possible results is a normal human characteristic. Only thing that would help you in lowering your stress related to this scenario is telling your self the following a few times.

'I am doing whatever is possible. Outcome is not in my hands. I would be able to carry on my life respectably irrespective of the results. So, WHY WORRY?'

Keep telling this to yourself whenever you feel anxiety over this scenario. You will notice a difference after telling it to yourself a few times.

Category 11

Problem 12:

What would happen to your family if you depart from this world early?

Suggested Approach:

This problem reminds me of a recent incident that happened in California, USA. The father, reported to have financial trouble shot dead his wife, his mother in law and three children. It somehow appears that he concluded that his family would not be able to survive without him. What a stretch of negative imagination! How much financial stress led him to commit this unthinkable crime, only he could tell. But this definitely tells that such thoughts, as the problem states must be handled timely.

World is not going to end with you. If you believe in God, you must also believe in the saying "Everyone in this world is born with his/her own destiny. Breadwinner is only a conduit thro' whom God provides to fulfill the destiny of the child". If God decides to remove that conduit, He would provide for an alternative. In any case the child would receive his due as per his destiny.

Let us also look around and see whether this is a real problem. You might know more than one family whose breadwinner departed from this world prematurely. How many members of those families you know could not survive? Each of them, you might have noticed, survived, and even in some cases turned out to be better achiever.

So the point is that it is only in your mind that you are indispensable to your family because at present you have taken all the responsibilities, big and small, on yourself. You cannot picture somebody else in your family being able to do the same. Nature's law is that it does not like vacuum or imbalance. In case the breadwinner is gone, responsibility would pass on and taken up by next competent member of the family. One also underestimates his family member's capabilities which they themselves did not know before they were put in the situation of handling it. It is the survival instinct that brings out the best of us in times of need.

Category 12

Problem 13:

You were expecting to get a promotion this fall, but some junior employee was promoted over you.

Suggested Approach:

There is no reason for you not to feel bad, particularly if it was due to some favoritism display. But question is whether now your reacting to it or just getting upset is going to help the matters. If you think there is a proper way to challenge this promotion, go ahead with it. Otherwise don't cause yourself more harm by taking stress because of it.

In 'Hindu' religion, there is a revered holy book named 'Shreemad Bhagwad Gita'. One of the main advices given therein by Lord Krishna is that most of the problems arise because of expectations. It says that you could have bliss only if you could control your expectations. It goes on to say that 'One should do his duties without expecting the results. If one is doing his duties selflessly, results are bound to follow on their own'.

Whether you follow that philosophy or not, let these expectations not spoil your present at least.

Category 13

Problem 14:

You wished from childhood to own a Bentley car but so far there appears no chance of that.

Suggested Approach:

In fact this is a self-created problem. This is something like 'Oh, I don't have any problem. Let me create one'.

Having high ambitions are good, but the bad part starts when we try to set ambitions without relating it to the ground realities. It is also harmful, further, to really expecting to achieve those even if one is not able to create any resources to meet those ambitions, though normally that person is doing better than most. In such cases, the opportunity of feeling good for your successes is overrun by this unrealistic ambition. Setting higher ambitions are fruitful only if after using all your strengths and resources, you are able to enjoy whatever level you could achieve. If one can't do that, such ambitions invariably lead to stressful situations.

This is not to say that being ambitious is bad. In fact, life would be very boring without ambitions. At the same time life would be very difficult if our ambitions are unrealistic. In cases of unrealistic scenarios, though one has achieved more because of higher ambitions, it might keep hurting not to have achieved the set goal.

To illustrate this point better, let us assume that you set goal at level 9. Let us also assume that without setting target you would have achieved goal of 4 and that your true potential is goal of 7. Now because you set your goal at 9 and you could achieve 7 is a good thing. It becomes bad only when you are not happy on achieving goal 7 because you could not achieve the set goal of 9, which to start with was unrealistic goal.

You can see how ambitions could help you or hurt you.

If you realize this and are happy with the results you achieve, you are already happy (stress gone!).

Category 14

Problem 15:

It has been found in various studies that people living simple lives were overall happier than the ones leading sophisticated life styles.

Likewise people paying more attention to customs connected to their religious festivals (like Xmas) were happier than those thinking about gifts for those occasions.

Suggested Approach:

You would be surprised to see the following example of inadvertent creation of ambitions which for many bring undesirable results.

Have you ever thought that even watching TV for some could result ultimately in stressful situations? Yes, it could definitely do that. When you watch TV, you are always presented with beautiful and handsome people wearing choicest clothes and using costliest available gadgets. Similarly you are presented the benefits of latest consumer items making latest fashion statements. Sometimes inner you start wishing to emulate or acquire even when you don't need that item and even when many might not be financially able to do that. That desire if unfulfilled could leave you with some unnoticed discomfort. The one, who tries to fulfill this desire without sufficient financial backing, could also face stress due to financial implications.

Chapter 6

Stress Releasers- part I

We have talked about the potential stress creators. Now let us try to look at stress releasers. There could be many types of stress releasers defined and selected differently by every one affected. Each stress releaser would not produce same results for every one. Every body has different impact from the same event. Let me explain a bit of memory, rather fading of memory. As you know fading of memory is a blessing for the human kind so graciously bestowed upon us by the Almighty. Take the instance of death of a near one. If this remains as live and as fresh in your mind as on the day of the event, you would be feeling as pathetic and distressed today as you were feeling on that day. Subsequent tragic events would further keep adding to our woes. That could make your life a living hell. But, that's not what happens in your daily life. That shows that all tragic and pleasant events go to the back of your mind. And that's the point I am trying to make. The tragic events become less bothering as time passes. With time, these start getting lower priority and keep gradually fading with respect to your day-to-day needs and activities. This all happens in a natural way designed in such a way that life could go on smoothly. But you might know some people who are not blessed with this natural phenomenon. Such people keep remaining hysteric long after the event. That means different people handle events of same magnitude in tragedy in different ways producing different results.

This chapter is meant to rationally guide you to have a handle on potential stress that could be caused by so many things. Believe me, if you could be successful in handling stress, not only you would improve your chances of being healthier, you would also be able to better handle the problems those gave you stress in the first place.

Let me explain this point. You might have watched sometimes Tennis Grand Slam Final match on TV. Usually the commentator would say, "At this point, it is a game as much of skill as much as a game of nerves". World number one player would suddenly make a double fault at some critical stage of the game. What does it say to you? The players are very conscientious of the stress of imagining 'If I fail'. Take the stress out of any player; his level of game would go much higher. Let me remind. Here we are talking of bad stress only that arises from the negative feeling of 'If I fail'! Good type of stress might have helped those players to reach where they are.

This is a typical example proving the existence and impact of good stress and bad stress. In this specific example, it is good type of stress that ignited the will in the player to reach at the top. But when this bad stress in the negative form of 'If I fail' creeps in his mind, his performance starts faltering. So holding the nerve also could mean to avoid the bad stress.

I have divided stress releasers in two broad parts: part I and part II.

Whereas part I would have all stress releasers that are only mentally handled by individuals in their own suitable way, part II is a well documented technique adopted and practiced in a specific way by all. In part II you would learn the relevant techniques of 'YOGA'.

Let us start with the stress releasers grouped in part I. You have to pick one or more depending on your own preferences and requirements.

1. The Master Key

This is the '**one fits all**' type of stress releaser. As pointed out earlier, stress is not something material. It lies in your mind. So it would be very logical to say that its solution also lies in your mind. Put another way, I could say that '**it is all in your head**'. Though this may not be completely true, but practically it is very close to that.

Remember '**the things change if you change the way you look at them**'?

The expression 'Treat others as you would like others to treat you' reinforces it further. It asks you to look at your action from others' perspective.

Related Scenario:

Most of the times when you have disagreement with others, it is probable that you are not trying to deal the topic from other person's angle. If you could do that, chances are that you would find some justification in his/her argument.

Let us take this example. You are working for a manufacturing company. The client rejected some of the products produced under your supervision. Your employer punishes you by imposing some penalty. You are feeling enraged. Your argument is 'I did my best with available facilities. Moreover, quality department should have checked before dispatch. My employer is totally unreasonable'. With these thoughts you might curse other management personnel too. You might bring this rage to your home. You might even think to take a negative approach in future production.

Try to put yourself in the shoes of the employer. What would have you done on receiving complaints or rejected material from your client? Your company's revenue and image was at stake. Would have you ignored it? If not, what would have you done? You might have tried to find, to your best judgment, the person responsible for this and would have taken some action so as to avoid this situation in future. You possibly might have imposed different punishment, but everyone is different with different capabilities to judge.

Once you do this, you would find your anger diluted. Possibly you might start thinking to find a way to improve the products. You might be more cautious about the quality of your product. You might even start interacting more with other departments to improve your product.

This difference was possible because you changed your way to look at it.

Take another instance. A teenager feels that he is being nagged when his mom tells him daily to drive carefully or to come home early. He sees it from a negative angle. He feels anger towards his mom. For a moment imagine that he looks at his mom's advice from a different angle. If he could think like 'how much my mom cares for my safety that she keeps thinking about me even when my response to that is so rough. She makes it a point to be at the door to see me off and remind me about my safety everyday. She always wishes me to be out of harms way and wants me reach home safely. How much she loves me!'

Again, just changing the way to look at the same event but with positive frame of mind, produced totally contrasting results. He would feel so happy about his mom's concern. For sure his mom would be happier than him.

I think you could see the contrast in results just by changing the way that kid looked at his mom's concerns.

Try to apply this approach to so many incidents you come across everyday. You would always see the difference when you look at them positively.

I think you could see the contrast in results just by changing the way that kid looked at his mom's advice.

If you could master the art of changing the way you look at the things, I believe you won't really need to use the other stress releasers much.

2. Be Practical

Next best approach to reduce stress is to have 'hands-on' approach. There would be lot of scenarios in which the best and only approach is to be practical. Some scenarios would have a solution with a plan and in some cases you have just to bear with it. Remember the instance under 'Finance Category' in Chapter 5? That example required a practical solution. There may be other scenarios where nothing could be done to change the situation. In such cases our approach again has to be practical.

Related Scenario:

Whenever there is a problem, ask from self, "Can I do something about it"? If answer is 'yes', then ask how and make a detailed plan to handle the problem. By telling yourself that something could be done takes your thoughts towards planning and executing instead of worrying. Now you would be feeling positive about the problem because this plan gives a hope of doing something about the problem creating positive vibrations all around. While making this effort, your stress would already have taken back seat. It is like putting blanket on your stress and diverting your mental and physical resources towards something positive.

If the answer is 'no' then you have to take a philosophical approach to convince your mind about the futility of worrying about something not having any solution with you. Worrying or developing stress in such case only would make the things worse. Asking that question to yourself consciously makes you realize that you can't do anything about it. Anytime you feel stressed from the same problem, again ask the same question to yourself. That way you would feel better and then just relax and decide to cross the bridge when you come to it.

This approach works in many extreme cases.

- Death of a near one is devastating experience for anyone.

- Loss of job is a big blow.

- Splitting with spouse or a close friend is agonizing as well.

In many such situations, you can't do anything. By reminding yourself a few times that you can't do anything about it does help control your emotions and lowering your stress. Asking this question and answering it also prepares you mentally to move on. This is the only practical way to handle it.

3. Heavens would not fall

This is the third best approach to handle your stress by adopting the 'Heavens won't fall' attitude towards your problem. It is something like saying 'so what?' on any action when asked to justify. In a way by saying this you are telling your mind that whatever happens, heavens would stay in their place, meaning life would go on.

You can approach most of the problems with this attitude with successful results with reference to reducing stress. This actually prepares you mentally for the worst outcome. When you say 'So What?', you are telling yourself that its results don't make difference to you. So when you are prepared for the worst outcome, how anything related to that matter could bother you? This attitude would be very useful in very grave situations to make you behave normal or even positive and thus ensuring better results. Need not to say that your stress level also would be very manageable.

Related Scenario:

Let us take one of the worst scenarios.

In the recent past there were lot of lay offs by many companies. It was noticed that the persons who were laid off were not under that much stress as the ones with possible chances of being laid off. What does it mean? For those already laid off, the worst was over and now they were engaged in making future arrangements for getting employed or improving their qualifications to get another job. Though they were facing financial hardships, their mental and physical resources were being realigned to make efforts for getting new job. That's a constructive process bringing out best of you. So they did not have much time to feel stressed, rather their mind was masked from being stressed by the attention they were paying to constructive efforts. Not only they were having no time for bad stress, they were having challenges ahead thus creating good type of stress which was helpful to face the difficult situation ahead.

Those who were about to lose job (that's what they thought) were afraid of going to the situation of being jobless. But they were not able to do anything other than fearing. Not that they would not survive if laid off, but the fear in their mind was playing havoc in their lives. Had they adopted the attitude 'Heavens are not going to fall even if we lose our job. We would be able to come out stronger from that challenge', they would have been stronger mentally releasing the stress caused by fear. Same attitude could be described as 'so what' attitude. You can avoid many tense situations by just telling yourself 'so what?'

4. Try Some New Habits

If you keep doing whatever you have been doing, you would keep getting the results you had been getting. Come out of the hole. Give your life another chance. That would ensure new approach and self-evaluation. I would rather prefer everybody, irrespective of stress, should introspect himself/herself once every year. This could be done along with New Year resolutions you make every year. You should look at yourself and ask, "Whether there is any better way of doing whatever I had been doing?" Either you would feel better because you would be satisfied with what you were doing, or you would realize some of the 'undesirable things' you were doing and would think of changing for the better.

Related Scenario:

Many people get tense on their way to work because of traffic jam. It is quite natural to get tense particularly if you are getting late to work. This tension could also lead to some very hasty decision having the potential of leading to some accident. To avoid this tension, it is better to start for work from home early. For that you might have to change what you normally do in the morning. Best option is to get up earlier than you normally do giving yourself little extra time for driving. Not only you would have better relaxed driving, you would have an overall better feeling all day.

If you keep doing what you regularly do, results are not going to change. Same thing would apply to most of other things that you are not happy with.

5. Drop ego, accept your mistake

I am sure you already realize that there is nothing called free lunch. Here I am not referring to something material. What I am referring to is your ego. You could trade your ego with stress free conditions. Said differently you could lower your ego to lower your stress. In its simplest definition the ego is the concept of self that acts as barrier between one's own mind and the world.

Jesus, peace and blessings be upon him, also says John 3:3 "Unless a man is born a second time, he can not enter the kingdom of God." Mullah Sadra, the revered Persian Sufi master of the 17th century, explains the above saying as: "The first birth is from the womb of a woman, the second birth is from the womb of ego-senses. To be born again requires the transformation of the ego-personality." It is the 'I' we understand ourselves to be. The ego is conscience and, in many instances, controls how we think. Believe me, ego is the reason for many situations creating stress.

It is our ego that doesn't allow you to accept your mistake. Once you accept your mistake, you would make efforts in the right directions to solve the problem. Accepting your mistake is the first step to diagnose any problem.

Of course, that does not mean you should not have any ego. Ego to the extent of maintaining self-respect is good and required for every human being. Even animals display the existence of ego. What is referred to here is ego associated with adamancy, arrogance and close-mindedness.

Related Scenario:

This part of our personality is very important for retaining our self. At the same time too much of it leads to so many problems. It is identified with 'I', 'Me' or 'Mine'. In our daily life this 'I' could lead to unnecessary unpleasant situations. If you start thinking like:

'I am senior to this person, why did he not greet me in the morning?'

'I am her husband. Why my wife did not take my permission before going to her parent's house'?

'I am his wife. Why did he not care to consult me before making this program'?

'This store clerk is not giving me proper respect. Does he not know who I am'?

Each one of you could easily relate to more than one such situation in your routine life where ego might have spoiled the relations between friends, relatives, coworkers and even spouses. Ego never allows you to accept your mistake. When any discussion turns into argument, rest assure it is ego that is playing dominant role. The persons involved in arguments are not having open mind to understand the other person's point of view. While one of them is speaking, most probably, the other one is thinking hard to counter the point.

Many investors lost money in the market crash of 2000. The story is being repeated in 2008. Main reason for an individual to lose lot of money in stocks is his/her ego. 'I made a decision to buy this stock. How could my decision be wrong? Now if I sell it at a loss, that would mean I was wrong in buying this stock. How could I be wrong? I can't make a mistake! I can prove it by holding the stock long enough for it to come back. When it would bounce back, every body else would be proven wrong and I would be right.' Here you see the instance and results of not accepting mistake because of inflated ego. On the other hand, the ones who were not under such influence of ego realized their mistake early and got out, cutting down their losses. These bear markets hurt investors more with ego problem.

Ego has spoiled many family unions. Everyday you could see this phenomenon playing in many homes. We can't take rejection easily, again because of ego. Treating rejection as illusion (in point# 9) could help us achieve much more. Any successful salesman could tell you that. You have to have subtle balance between ego and self-respect.

If you really don't want stress, dropping ego and accepting your mistakes would go a long way in helping you manage your stress.

6. Be a giver

Conflicts start when you try to get a little more out of others. When you try to give a little more to those around you, you become happy and successful. Many a times giving is not sacrifice, giving is success. Giving does not have to be materially providing something; it could be providing kind words and physical help. A small act of kindness spreads happiness all around. Any act of kindness brings joy to whole environment. Joy, happiness and success is a sure stress buster.

Related Scenario:

This is another beautiful way of getting joy and peace to your mind. Lot of situations involve conflict of interest.

Have you come across a leader who has been elected to high office? If you look back at his history of younger age, chances are good that he used to be involved in community events. At that time that young man was not trying to get more out of others, rather he was trying to give little more. He was making sacrifices for others, may be, not for the sake of sacrifice. May be he was making sacrifice for success or may be, he was genuinely trying to help those in need. Whatever may be the intention, success followed him because of that approach of giving.

You would come across many business owners going out of way to please customers. Their object is not spreading happiness around; they recognize that giving to others is a path to success.

Sale events are organized not to benefit customers though the items are made available at lower price than their original price. That approach they employ again for success.

That is not to say that making sacrifice always leads to reduction of stress. Sometimes making sacrifice could lead to higher stress if sacrifice is always linked to returns and expectations. If sacrifice is made without any expectations in return, it gives immense joy to the giver and receiver. This makes you happy because you get the feeling of being useful to somebody. The receiver is happy because he gets the feeling of kindness from somebody. In fact it has been systematically measured that there are more than just the giver or the receiver who are happy. Even the person who is watching the act of kindness in operation also gets equal sense of joy as the giver and receiver gets. Is it not a really win-win situation for everybody? Of course it reduces stress of all involved.

7. Forgive

Somebody treated you or your loved one in unfair way. You want that person to be punished for that act. And you want that to be done at whatever cost. You are right. That's human. Justice must be done. But if it takes time for that justice to come, what goes in your mind? A sense of anger! Revengeful mood! You had already lost because of unfair treatment. Now all the time you are losing your peace of mind. That is now additional loss.

Like other problems, let's look at it from another angle. Is it possible that the offender had no intention of hurting you, or may be he is very remorseful for his act. Whether any of the damage could be undone by punishing this person? Most of all, is it under your control to punish that person? I know that it is very difficult to think from this angle. But for a moment for the sake of realizing what I want to say, could you try to imagine the resultant scenario if you forgive this person? Whether it is your spouse cheating on you or your son's arrogant behavior, think for a minute if you could forgive. Does it bring any feeling of relative peace to your mind? You would instantly realize the power of forgiveness. You could find a big difference in the state of your mind before and after forgiving.

Forgiveness is a very powerful tool tried by many people in total mess, especially when justice was taking long time to come. It is for nothing that our religious books always teach us to forgive the sinner.

I want you to remember that you are not forgiving the sinner for his/her benefit. You are doing it to relieve yourself from the agony you had been experiencing from your revengeful desire. Now that is separate output that, because of this act of forgiveness of yours, the sinner also benefits by having less guilt on his/her mind or with the sense of being pardoned. We are not talking about his/her benefits, but here we are talking about you. By forgiving the sinner, you are able to put an end to the sense of agony you were experiencing right from the time of the incident. After pardoning that person you are mentally able to close that chapter and move forward. With the closing of this chapter goes your agony and stress associated with that.

Related Scenario:

The concept of forgiveness and reconciliation are preached by all religions. Famous personalities in history have sought to adopt this act. Well known instances include:

- Mahatma Gandhi forgave his assassin.

- Nelson Mandela forgave his captors who kept him in jail for 27 years.

- Pope John Paul II made peace with the man who tried to kill him and was serving jail time for that.

The most recent case is that of Priyanka Gandhi, daughter of former Prime Minister of India, Rajiv Gandhi. A suicide bomber killed Mr. Rajiv Gandhi in 1991. Ms. Nalini Murugan, who was charged to be implicit in the case, was convicted to life imprisonment. It was in 2008, after 17 years, that Priyanka Gandhi sought meeting with the killer in prison cell, possibly for calming her turbulent thoughts she was troubled with for such a long time. Though nothing was announced to the media, Nalini is quoted to have expressed as if she had been pardoned.

These cases demonstrate the healing powers of simple act of forgiveness.

8. Have faith in yourself

'I can do it' approach not only helps you in making big achievements in life, it immensely helps you in successfully implementing stress- relieving techniques.

If the problem that was source of your stress is gone, stress would also be gone. It has also been stated that the problem is handled much better with reduced stress. That might look like a catch-22 position. To come out of this situation, there is another way. Have faith in yourself. Always feel the confidence that you have the capability of doing it. That confidence engages the brain in constructive direction thus blanketing your stress. You are able to handle the problem in more efficient way because your stress is no longer playing the hindering role. Better results follow for your problem and your stress.

Related Scenario:

It won't need a specific example to illustrate this obvious point. Any body could achieve nothing if he did not have confidence of doing it. Many people in their daily lives demonstrate this. Do you think Michael Phelps could have won 8 Gold Medals In 2008 Olympics if he did not have faith in himself?

All big achievers have one thing in common. They have faith in their capabilities to achieve.

9. Treat rejection as illusion

Rejection word itself sounds insulting. That could be the reason we don't like somebody to reject our offer or suggestion.

Related Scenario:

Let's consider it this way. You make a suggestion or offer to somebody because you want a specific thing to happen. You have no means to know whether the person whom you are making that suggestion would also want it to happen. You won't know that until you make that suggestion to him. There are chances that he might like it or may be he won't like it. If he does not like it, he would refuse. This communication from him that he did not like it is interpreted as rejection and you start feeling bad. Is it a good reason to feel bad? What if he would have accepted it? But that acceptance chance won't happen if you don't ask in the first place. First scenario of his not accepting keeps the situation unchanged. So when nothing is changed because of your making suggestion, what did you lose? Did any thing change from what it was before you made the suggestion? Therefore his rejecting your idea did not result in any loss, and therefore treating rejection as bad is only an illusion. But result of 2nd scenario of his acceptance would make you feel happy because that is what you wanted to happen.

Let's see it this way. You are at level 3. You want to go to level 5. For that you need someone's help. You asked a few people. Let us assume that all of them refused. You are still at level 3. You did not lose. The fear of rejection you had did not bring any negative result as far as your level is concerned. That means that fear was only an illusion.

But practically, there would be somebody who would help. You will find that person only by asking a few people. But if you are scared of refusal (rejection) you would never meet the guy who would have eventually helped and your chances of going to level 5 are zero. By asking you are creating chances of something happening that you want to happen.

If you had not asked, you would have continued to be at level 3 not knowing whether by asking you could have achieved level 5. That thought of 'not knowing' could be a continuous source of stress. By asking, irrespective of the result, you at least came out of the state of 'not knowing'. You would be satisfied with the thought that you did whatever was possible. Thus you are able to avoid the scenario of a thought 'had I asked, may be I could have succeeded'. That removes a source of prolonged stress.

Never fear rejection. Further never get depressed because of rejection that might turn out to be a stepping-stone to your success. Success is a very important tool to bring joy and reduce stress.

Chapter 7

Stress Releasers- part II (YOGA)

Apart from the stress releasers discussed earlier and illustrated with different scenarios, this practice is a great proven way to be at peace with self not only when you have stress, rather all the time. It is something like preventive maintenance and not breakdown maintenance. This position of being at peace all the time is achievable through time tested 'way of life' known as YOGA. Why is it called 'way of life' and not exercise? The reason is that yoga does not just provide benefits for your physical well being, it provides you with total benefits - physical, mental, spiritual, flexibility, vitality and overall wellbeing. This technique is especially useful when other stress releasers are not working adequately because of the nature of the source of stress.

This is useful for everybody irrespective of his/her stress levels.

In this chapter you would learn some techniques those are part of a well-documented practice of 'YOGA' adopted and practiced since ancient times with unparalleled benefits. The techniques we would chose in this lesson will be those which I consider most relevant to manage stress though these would bring you many other benefits as well.

A brief introduction to yoga would be helpful here. Yoga has been practiced for centuries in South East Asian countries by learned saints or yogis (probably yoga word is derived from that or may be yogi is derived from yoga). It is a proven technique and I can personally vouch for its stress releasing/managing effectiveness based on my personal experience. Yoga is a conscious process of total health development technique aimed at physical, mental, psychological, intellectual, emotional and spiritual uplifting. It can be classified into four classes:

- *Karma Yoga* (work)

- *Bhakti Yoga*   (worship)

- *Gnana Yoga*   (philosophy)

- *Raja Yoga*   (psychic control)

Each of this class is good and compliments others in the class. The class of relevance here is 'Raja Yoga' – method of self-control. This teaches us to control various inner forces at physical and psychological levels to reach a state of freedom. Raja Yoga is further classified into different classes like

- *Yama*

- *Niyama*

- *Asana*

- *Pranayama*

- *Dharna*

- *Dhyana*

- *Samadhi,* etc.

Each of these could be further differentiated into external and internal methods of control.

Adoption of these methods will not only be instrumental in releasing stress, it would condition your body so that your body could adopt it as a 'way of life' and you could manage your stress in all conditions.

For achieving maximum benefits of bringing peace to your mind along with other physical benefits, I would recommend practicing

- Three *pranayama kriyas,* and

- *Shavasana* (corpse pose)

Before starting I would like to remind you that I would limit our exposure to Yoga mostly as is relevant to releasing stress, though you would receive other immense benefits as well. In general we would call these *asanas* as relaxation exercises.

Instructions to start:

First of all, go through all instructions thoroughly and understand the procedure before starting to perform. Though these *asanas* and *kriyas* are very light and beneficial for everybody, you are advised to talk to your physician about the personal suitability. Important instructions as to when to do and what precautions you should take are briefed hereunder.

Perform these *asanas/kriyas*

- empty stomach in the morning, or

- 4-6 hours after meals, or

- 2 hours after liquid drinks.

- After attending to morning natural call.

- In lose attire.

- On a soft mat (not cushioned).

- Followed by complementing *asana* where applicable.

Do not

- Perform these *asanas/kriyas* if you are pregnant or during female monthly periods or other serious ailments.

- Force your body to attain perfect posture. Try to achieve only to the extent your body allows you without strain. Your achievement degree would improve with time.

- Expose yourself to cold air or cold bath immediately after performing these *asanas*. Give 10 – 15 minutes gap.

- Breathe through mouth. Try breathing through nose.

For performing recommended *asanas/kriyas* you would need to dress in a lose attire. You would also need a soft mat (not cushioned) of 3'X6' size and a fairly ventilated room. In case your home is centrally conditioned, it would help to open a window or door for about 2 – 3 minutes to bring fresh air into the room.

You would also do some warm up exercises before starting *asanas/ kriyas* for opening up your body organs. This warm up need not be long. You may simply walk briskly over treadmill or have a few small jumps in the air while keeping your arms and shoulders lose and in symmetric motion.

Pranayam:

Pranayam is derived from the word '*pran*' which is Sanskrit word meaning force of life. All different forms of *pranayam* involve controlled breathing, breathing air being part of '*pran*'. The classical definition of *pranayam* describes it to be control of vital life force and is achieved by changing the rhythm and control of inhalation and exhalation process. While you breathe in (inhale), you are bringing oxygen from the atmosphere into your system. Many of our organs require oxygen to create energy and for other biological processes. When you breathe out (exhale), you are getting rid of toxins and wastes like carbon monoxide, carbon dioxide and other trace gases. Breathing provides vital living force to the body, and the only center it could be controlled and harnessed is respiratory system. Three *kriyas* of *pranayam* I would like you to practice are;

- *Kapal Bhati*

- *Bahmya Pranayam*

- *Aum vilom* also known as *nadi shudhikaran*

Procedures:

Sit down on the mat in lotus pose. Pull heel of your left leg as close and on to your right thigh as comfortably possible and put heel of right leg on the top of left leg thigh. If you are not feeling comfortable doing this just put one heel on opposite thigh and the other one as close as possible. You may sit in some other comfortable pose also if this pose does not suit you. You could even sit on a chair and perform these *kriyas*. During these *kriyas*, keep your torso straight, head straight and shoulder going in line with pushed out chest. Your knees should be near ground as much as comfortably possible. Back of your hands should rest on your knees while forefinger and thumb touching each other at the tips giving it shape of a circle. Other three fingers of your hands should be just straight open.

Kapalbhati Pranayam:

This mainly is – active exhalation and slow inhalation exercise.

Procedure:

- Exhale with a burst – push your breath outside with a little jerk to abdominal diaphragm and lungs.

- Only abdominal muscles move while other parts like shoulders and face remain stationary.

- Inhale slowly, involuntarily, naturally, having a feeling of achievement.

- While exhaling, think that you are pushing out toxins and negative energy.

- There is no time gap between the inhaling and exhaling process.

- Keep a calm posture throughout, especially your facial muscles.

- Concentrate on your naval point.

Do this cycle 20 to 30 times.

- Do this exercise for 2 to 3 minutes, never more than 5 minutes.

- Whenever you feel tired, take a little break until you are breathing normally.

- Don't exert any excessive pressure.

Benefits:

- Takes out stress and depression.

- Improves prostrate problem.

- Helps people with constipation problem.

- Reduces obesity.

Bahmya Pranayam:

Bahmya Pranayam should follow *Kapaal Bhati pranayam*. It should be performed for 4 to 5 times.

Procedure:

- Exhale completely followed by pushing the remnant air in your lungs and diaphragm with a little burst. Air should be felt passing through your throat with a little hissing sound.

- Keep the breath out as long as comfortably possible.

- While keeping the breath outside make effort to bring your chin close to your chest.

- Push back your abdomen towards your back as much as comfortably possible.

- Keep calm on your face.

- Keep your posture straight.

- Keep your arms stretched and resting on your knees.

- When you can't hold your breath any longer, inhale slowly without sudden rush. Let your lungs and abdomen fill with air.

- While inhaling, have a feeling of absorption and achievement like your body is getting something very nutritious.

- Repeat the above process when your breathing becomes normal. When tired take a little break.

- Do it any where between 1 to 10 times. Maximum limit is 20.

Benefits:

It has all the benefits of *Kapaal Bhati* described above. The benefits related to prostrate, obesity and constipation further improve. Helps throw toxins and tunes up internal system. Brings grace to your skin and face.

Aum Vilom (Nadi Shudhikaran):

This is perhaps the simplest form of *Pranayam*. This basically is breathing - exhaling and inhaling - alternately through left and right nostrils. That cleans our body's nerves, nerve centers and body channels. Inhaling through clean system provides our body more oxygen and helps to excrete toxins in efficient way. That is very useful for body and mind.

Procedure:

- Raise your right hand. Press the flap of your right nostril to close it with the help of your thumb leaving other fingers open and extended but not apart. Rest part of your hand should be pointing upwards near your forehead.

- Inhale deeply and slowly through your left nostril.

- After inhaling is complete, hold your breath and close your left nostril with the ring finger of your same hand. Leave other fingers of your hand extended in a way that your thumb is pointing upward near your forehead.

- Exhale slowly through your right nostril.

- After exhaling is over, start inhaling from the same nostril (right nostril) while pressing your left nostril with your ring finger.

- After inhaling is over through right nostril, press and close your right nostril with the thumb of your same hand (right hand).

- Exhale slowly through your left nostril.

- That completes one cycle.

- Complete 5 to 10 cycles in this manner.

Benefits:

In addition to the benefits provided by *Kapaal Bhati*, this *kriya* cleanse your system better particularly nerve center thus being practically beneficial for all the functions of your body.

Shavasana (Corpse Pose):

This is very basic pose and is most important in relaxation techniques. Practically in this *asana* your target is to do nothing. That's why this is also called 'corpse pose'. But doing nothing is not easy. You have to go through a few steps to reach the stage of doing nothing.

Procedure:

- Lie down on your back.

- Toes of your feet should naturally fall outwards and little parted.

- Your arms should be resting besides your body with palms facing upwards.

- Your head should be naturally tilted on one side comfortably.

- Your eyes should be closed and relaxed.

- Your face should be calm with a smile.

- There should not be any tightness on your face. It should be relaxed.

- No part of your body should be tight. All parts should be loose, resting naturally and relaxed.

- Breathing should be normal but controlled. While you inhale, pay attention to your abdomen and chest going up. While exhaling, abdomen and chest go down. Exhaling time should be approximately double the inhaling time. You can regulate the timing by counting mentally.

- Tell your mind you are calm and peaceful.

- Intermittently scan your body mentally, from toes to head and from fingers to shoulders, checking that all parts are relaxed.

- Imagine yourself lying in an environment of your liking where you have felt most calm and joyful ever.

- Intermittently, pay attention to your breathing and parts of your body.

If you start feeling sleepy and feel totally relaxed while doing it, that would mean that you are doing it correctly.

After you have done it for 5 to 10 minutes, tilt your face upwards, make a cup with both your hands, place the cup on your eyes and slowly open your eyes to get these gradually accustomed to the light around. Get up. You are set for the day.

Benefits:

- This is used for complete recovery of energy after performing exercises.

- It improves your energy levels.

- It is most relaxing posture relieving you from all tension, stress, depression etc.

- If you felt fatigued during any posture or other exercises, it recoups energy to make you feel refreshed and takes away your exhaustion and tiredness.

- It elevates your inner consciousness about yourself and your parts of body, mentally and physically.

———

Chapter 8

Glass Is Half Full

Everybody must have heard this popular saying. Instead of saying 'look from a different angle', it says 'look from a positive angle'. Remember, 'Things change if you change the way you look at them'? Here we could improve that saying by changing it to 'Things change for the better if you look at them in a positive way'. This is another way to think positive. This approach is intricately embedded deeply throughout this book. As a matter of fact, it has been referred to in many of the stress releasers.

Any event could be looked upon from more than one angle. When you try to evaluate any event optimistically, you would get positive vibrations soothing your mind. Same event evaluated pessimistically would add to the stress by emitting negative vibrations.

If you analyze the incident narrated in Chapter 1 of this book, the message unmistakably is 'just think positive'. Baba Ji reminded my father about what he had (glass half full) and not to worry about what he did not have (glass half empty). My father was further reminded that loss of what he had would be bigger problem than the problems bothering him. He was reminded not to feel bothered with problems, rather to count his blessings. My father, without any material change in the circumstances or status of his problems, came home relieved. What was done? Just looking at the problems from the angle of 'glass half full'.

Each one of us could apply the same logic to our daily life.

At young age teens see the shortcoming of their parents. The only thing that dominates their mind with respect to mom is how she told them not to go out and play or how she chides them for not completing their schoolwork or when she asks them to go to bed early. They evaluate their father's love for them based only on the number of times he did not interfere with their activities. They never try to see the strengths of their parents. They don't like the tone in which sometimes their parents address them. The same 'irritants' or 'chiding' looked from a different angle could have become totally pleasant events. For a moment imagine, like in Chapter 6, that he looks at his mom's advice from a different angle. If he could think like 'how much my mom cares for my safety that she keeps thinking about me even when my response to that is so rough. She makes it a point to be at the door to see me off and remind me about my safety everyday. She always wishes me to be out of harms way and wants me reach home safely. How much she loves me!' Similarly he could find love in his dad's advices, if looked differently. As these teens grow and become parents themselves, they start realizing that the positive qualities and sacrifices their parents made for them far outweighed the irritants. But at that time they cannot turn the clock back.

Imagine the situation where the same teens realized the good point of their parents (glass half full) at their young age. Would they not make wonderful relations with their parents? Would those parents not have given to their kids even more? It could have been a win-win situation raising level of happiness all around. All this – just by thinking positively!

Terrorism is total contrast of positive thinking. It is just opposite to what we are talking about positive thinking. They see only that glass is half empty. That results in total lose-lose situation. That creates loss and anxiety for others resulting in lowering happiness all around.

This is mentioned just to point out the devastating results of negative thinking. Any young man could abort his endeavors of doing business thinking he does not have enough resources. Another person with same resources but positive frame of mind would try to find a way to find resources or try to modify his business plan with a total approach as to how to do it. The first type tried to find a reason for not doing a business. Second type tried to have the approach as to how to work out a plan. In second case, he at least created a chance to succeed whereas in first case the chance is zero.

Imagine a category of people you know in two groups. One, those are successful in life. Though there is no specific parameter for such division, for the sake of discussion, we would call them successful if they are overall happy. The most common trait you would notice in this category would be that for any problem they try to work at, 'how can I make it happen?' The second group would have in common the approach of finding a reason that why they can't do it.

That approach goes miles in producing desirable and undesirable results. Said the other way, your approach to life decides whether you lead a happy or unhappy life.

———————

Chapter 9

Hands-on Approach

When you carry unmanaged stress, it affects your life in many ways:

- It affects your family relations.

- You are not able to give your best at your work place.

- You can't concentrate on anything.

- Small events irritate you easily.

- Negative thoughts keep nagging your mind.

- You are more susceptible to diseases.

- Your immune system start losing strength.

- You try to find pleasure in external material world.

- You start having negative thoughts about whole world.

There are so many other potential problems you might face.

Every one would definitely like to get rid of the source of these problems, namely, stress.

Have you ever faced a situation where you feel uncomfortable about something but you can't place what it was? Many a times you just have a feeling of discomfort without being really aware of what is bothering you. There are many situations in day-to-day life where you want to get rid of these unnecessary teasing problems.

You could do it by a simple technique of making a list and handle the things in a systematic way. It sounds like too simple to be true, but you have to try it to see what I mean. It is almost same technique that I experienced in Chapter 1. Remember Baba Ji making a list of problems?

Here we will be a little different from the way the problem was solved in Chapter 1. Go through the following steps.

1. Make a list of all the stress contributing problems.

2. Rearrange this list in order of gravity of the problem, the least grave problem being first and the gravest problem being last.

3. Go over each problem one by one.

4. See if that problem could be handled with the help of available resources, including the techniques you learnt in this book. Note down your conclusions, including plan if any, against each of the problems.

5. If the answer to number 4 above is 'yes', include that problem in a second list.

6. Make a third list of the problems those you answered 'no' to number 4 above and for which you don't find any apparent solution.

7. Out of this third list identify and delete the problems that you think are not impacting your life much and with which you can live without doing anything.

8. Start taking action on the second list.

9. After finishing that list go to the third list.

10. Go over each problem one by one. Try to solve one problem at a time. At any given time, try to concentrate only on one problem.

Compare your stress level after the point number 7 above to the stress level you had before starting this exercise. I believe you would already be having much lower stress level than when you started. That would be because you have come out of the stage of uncertainty to the stage where you can quantify your problems. Chances are good that when you were going through this exercise, you were able to recognize the insignificance of some problems.

That being so, a major objective of this exercise is already met after you reached point number 8 above. You are already feeling much better. (I am so sure about this that I am ready to refund the face value of this book to you in case you are not feeling any better about your stress level at this point. In that unlikely scenario, please return this book with proof of price you paid within 60 days of the purchase mentioning the code "thanks, but no thanks". You can follow the instructions to follow on my website 'howibecamestressfree.com'.)

At this point you have 3 lists.

*   Original list having all the problems.

*   Second list where you feel the problems could be resolved by adopting certain plan.

- Third list where you feel that the problems don't have any apparent solution.

Please remember that the order of problems in these lists have to be in the ascending order of seriousness; least grave problem at the top and gravest problem at the bottom.

Here, keep in mind; you are trying to solve the problems for managing your stress and not finding absolute solutions to your problems. Of course removing the root cause of stress, that is your problems, would take away your stress too.

Now your mind is well aware of the problems and their status. There is no vagueness nagging your mind with uncertain, unknown problems. Now you are already constructively thinking of tackling those problems and you have a plan. Start executing your plan for the problems in the second list, one at a time. After you have solved some of the problems, your stress related to those problems would be already gone. Now you would be left with some unsolved problems in second list and problems in the third list. Here you have to try to manage stress related to these problems by adopting techniques described in this book in Chapter 6 and Chapter 7. If the stress releasers in Chapter 6 don't help you bring down your stress level, only course left with you is to try stress releaser of Chapter 7. Rest assure, practicing this technique is definitely going to be helpful within couple of weeks of starting it.

You could consult me by posting your problem on my web site www.howibecamestressfree.com.

You could send me email at joshi@howibecamestressfree.com. I would try to answer based on the information you provide and based on my best approach to handle that problem.

It is possible that, depending upon your progress of plan or some new developments, your level of stress again goes up. Repeat the above exercise. Of course this time, number of problems on your list is likely to be much smaller. Gradually you would reach a stage where you would be handling stress related to only recent problems. Practicing this process for at least 21 times would give a very fair chance to reach a stage where you could have a feeling of 'stress free' state, which, as I explained is the best state where you could handle your stress levels with most ease. Why this number 21? I believe, based on various sources, that it takes 21 repetitions for a habit to develop.

If you could combine the above stated practice with YOGA exercises detailed in Chapter 7, you would notice substantial improvement in your life in addition to easier handle on stress levels.

The purpose of the author in whole this effort is to add another person with minimum stress and positive outlook to this world resulting in elevating the **'happiness level of this world'**.